Hiatal Hernia Syndrome/Vagus Nerve Imbalance

The Most Common Health Syndrome In Mankind

With Illustrated Corrections, *Third Edition*

By Steven Rochlitz, PhD

Foreword by Howard Abens, D.C.

ISBN: 0-945262-61-9 72 pages, 15 Illustrations
$20.00 each. Shipping: $5.00. ($8.00 air mail to non-U.S.
countries.) Prices subject to change.

Steven Rochlitz, PhD
P.O. Box 2154
Cottonwood, Arizona 86326 USA
(928) 649-2116
www.wellatlast.com
info@wellatlast.com

Legal Disclaimer: This book is a theoretical discussion and is not intended to diagnose, treat, or prescribe for any medical condition. For this, consult your medical or health practitioner.

To

The Memory of

My Mother,

Jacqueline

Hiatal Hernia Syndrome/ Vagus Nerve Imbalance

The Most Common Health Syndrome In Mankind… and Womankind

With Illustrated Corrections

Third Edition

By Steven Rochlitz, PhD

Acknowledgement

I thank Dr. Howard Abens, who is also a seminar graduate of mine, for writing the foreword. It is fitting that it comes from a physician, who in his eighties, is still correcting hiatal hernias!

I am pleased that he has added some of the related techniques in this book, and has now provided his feedback on them.

Thanks also to Chris Curran, my lifeline to the outside world.

TABLE OF CONTENTS

Section I: The Nature of the HHS/VNI—Page 11

Section II: The Corrections—Page 37

Foreword

My name is Howard Abens, and I live in Osage, Iowa. I graduated from Palmer College of Chiropractic in 1957. I've been practicing Chiropractic for a little more than 55 years. It never ceases to amaze me that there is always something new to learn.

I first met Dr. Rochlitz at a seminar that he presented in Sioux Falls, South Dakota some twenty years ago. He is a very knowledgeable man, and I have a great deal of appreciation for him.

I have worked with hiatal hernia, diaphragm and esophagus problems for years, but never made the vagus nerve connection. This is a big plus, and so easy to do! Dr. Rochlitz does a great deal of research and study for which I am very thankful.

Before this, I never even considered hiatal hernia to be a problem in babies or young people…but now I am finding that it is quite common. Being able to detect it and correct it is a big advantage.

This book is so beneficial in helping to detect and correct problems with vagus nerve, hiatal hernia, diaphragm, trigger points for the lungs and heart, and for sleep apnea and swallowing. It is also helpful in the areas of information about diet and lifestyle changes that are beneficial to overall health.

This book uniquely contains the interconnectedness of vagus nerve imbalance, heart problems, sleep apnea, hiatal hernia, breathing difficulties, food allergies, the esophagus, GERD/reflux, anxiety or panic attack, asthma, and even the more recent problems of multiple chemical sensitivities (MCS) and electromagnetic sensitivities (EMFS)…working with all these aspects is so beneficial in helping the patient to live a more normal and healthy life.

Thank you, Dr. Rochlitz.

Dr. Howard Abens
Osage, IA
September, 2012

Preface To The Third Edition

A new edition to this book was necessary for several reasons. The text was revised, an index was added, as was an important section on the nature, testing and treatment options for sleep apnea. In 2012, even cancer has been found to be linked to sleep apnea—itself linked often to the Hiatal Hernia Syndrome.

I have also received a foreword to this book from Dr. Howard Abens.

I hope these additions are appreciated.

Steven Rochlitz, PhD
Arizona
September, 2012

Preface

The genesis of this book goes back to a lengthy article I wrote in 2002. For years, my readers had asked me for a separate book on the Hiatal Hernia Syndrome/Vagus Nerve Imbalance with illustrated corrections. Here it is. This book remains the only one to link the HHS/VNI with both hidden deeper problems, in some people, and with such results as sleep apnea, asthma, and heart problems. It is with great difficulties that these works of mine have been written or rewritten.

There is more on the possible relationship of the HHS/VNI to underlying problems in my book, *Porphyria: The Ultimate Cause of Common, Chronic or Environmental Illnesses. With Diet, Supplement and Energy Balancing.* It is hoped that the reader will get and read "the whole picture" at some point. But I realize that some people cannot wait to get the crucial information contained herein.

Now you can get started with self-help corrections. Just be careful, and be gentle with yourself. Please realize that these are the basic corrections. There are many other things that 32 years experience has taught me. Nonetheless the information, and methods, in this book should be—*and have been*—of immense value to the sufferers of the HHS. Make sure to make the diet and lifestyle corrections also contained in this book. There are many *things to do, not just to read.*

For the second edition I added numerous techniques, which are related to the correction of the Hiatal Hernia.

Steven Rochlitz, PhD
Arizona
December, 2011

Section I

The Nature of

The Hiatal Hernia Syndrome

and

Vagus Nerve Imbalance

12

Hiatal Hernia Syndrome/Vagus Nerve Imbalance

The Hiatal Hernia Syndrome, with Vagus Nerve Imbalance, may be the most common set of complaints in our species. Probably most people who are chronically unwell have this syndrome. Here we will first see what the Hiatal Hernia is, and then look at the possible symptoms that can arise from this syndrome, and its associated Vagus Nerve Imbalance. Then we will discuss many things to do that can improve this syndrome. This will culminate in depicting some techniques to get the stomach to go back down, and to restore balance to the Vagus Nerve, and the diaphragm.

Figure 1. Hiatal Hernia—above the diaphragm, where it doesn't belong. See also the front cover.

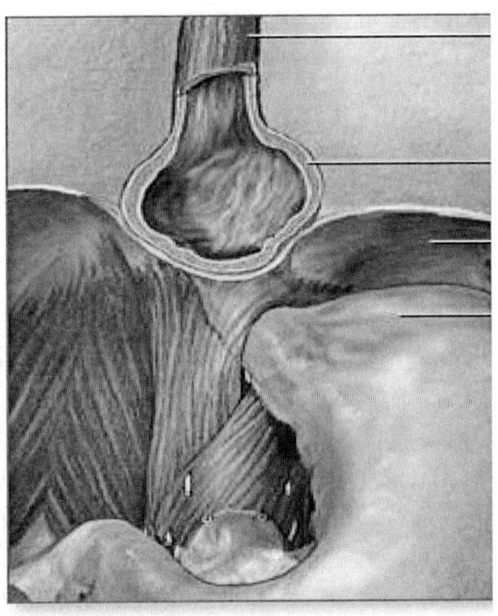

Esophagus

Hiatal Hernia

Diaphragm

Upper stomach (aka the fundus)

Note, that in Fig. 1, the cutaway portion of the stomach has gone up through the diaphragm, and is now above it. Wellness can return if, and when, that part of the stomach goes—and stays—below the originally small, diaphragmatic opening.

This can take some doing, in some cases. Many things may be involved, as we shall see. It often requires learning a set of techniques far beyond the simple "pull down" some perform.

Make sure to understand the abbreviations used here. **HHS** will stand for Hiatal Hernia Syndrome. **VNI** will stand for Vagus Nerve Imbalance. Many people may have had this problem for much of their lives, and it only keeps getting worse. It may eventually cause or exacerbate serious heart and/or lung disease in some. I hypothesize that it is deeply involved in many chronic conditions, *and* in acute porphyria attacks, and in MCS, EMFS, and in having food "allergies", asthma, and sleep apnea.

Both mainstream and alternative medicine seem to be unaware or unappreciative of the serious illness or suffering the HHS commonly causes. It can cause any of the visceral organs to malfunction. By late middle age, 50-85% of the population has this undetected condition. This factor may even be a predictor of life expectancy, as we shall see.

The biochemist Carey Reams, PhD, said, "illness begins with the Vagus Nerve." The Hiatal Hernia Syndrome (HHS), by pinching the Vagus Nerve, causes Vagus Nerve Imbalance (VNI). However, one may have hidden, underlying illness(es) that *already* have disordered the Vagus Nerve! The Vagus Nerve could be imbalanced from heavy metal excess (lead, arsenic, mercury, other), or porphyria[1], or any malady that affects the nervous system. (Twenty percent of mankind has a hidden porphyria genetic defect—it is *not* a rare disease.) This imbalance is often a hyperexcitability, but a decreased energy state is also possible. In a Hiatus Hernia, or Hiatal Hernia, the upper portion of the stomach protrudes through the opening (hiatus) in the diaphragm, as in Fig. 1.

Theodore Baroody, D.C. called the Hiatal Hernia Syndrome, "the Mother of All Illness," and he stated that nearly "every [noninfectious] condition [except trauma] is the direct result of some digestive dysfunction."[2] He wrote that the Hiatal Hernia Syndrome is "dangerous and brings about constant imbalances that lead to all maladies known to mankind." He found that over 85% of his patients, when tested, have a Hiatal Hernia. I, of course, have found, that for some people, several underlying problems cause the HHS/VNI itself, making them the "Grandmother" of chronic illness.

My own clients have included many with fatigue/fibromyalgia and/or food, chemical, and electromagnetic sensitivities. They have the Hiatal Hernia Syndrome over 90% of the time. It's no coincidence. I cannot blame the reader for any initial disbelief, but 29 years of working on this problem in people has made the matter clear to me. Seemingly unrelated illnesses, or symptoms, can often immediately be relieved when "the stomach is brought down," and/or the Vagus Nerve is re-balanced.

Below is a list of symptoms from the HHS and/or VNI. I am not saying the HHS/VNI is the sole cause of each of these complaints or conditions. Sometimes it exacerbates a condition, and other elements are involved. Let's look at how the Hiatal Hernia and Vagus Nerve Imbalance can cause so many complaints and organ problems. Later we will see how to make some corrections for the Hernia, the Vagus Nerve, and the diaphragm. The corrections can last for years in some people, or only for seconds in others.

One difficulty in seeing all this clearly, by the standard medical profession, often arises because many factors can prevent the stomach from "going back down" or "staying down." My own improved techniques, in this next section, may make this change last longer, and thus the improvement in these many seemingly, unrelated conditions is observable.

I have also found that a hidden heart defect that one out of three people have—the PFO (Patent Foramen Ovale)—is deeply linked to the HHS/VNI. This may be one reason why only some with the HHS suffer so much, and others with it do not. I would advise anyone with the Hiatal Hernia who is prone to arrhythmia, tachycardia, bradycardia, hypertension, orthostatic hypotension, or fainting, to get tested for the PFO.[3] [See my separate "sister" book on the PFO, if you have cardiac symptoms.]

You can get the TransCranial Doppler test to look for the PFO. It is also possible that other underlying heart problems are closely and adversely affected by the HHS/VNI. I have observed that angina, leaky valves, atrial fibrillation, supraventricular tachycardia, and other heart problems, can all become "active" due to the effects of the HHS/VNI. So it can be crucial for anyone with any heart condition to find out if s/he has the HHS/VNI.

Possible Symptoms of Vagus Nerve Imbalance/Hiatal Hernia Syndrome

- Panic Attack
- Shortness of breath, gasping
- Tachycardia, bradycardia, heart conditions
- Palpitations
- Belching
- Bloating
- Gas
- Anxiety
- Hypertension or Hypotension
- Asthma (may be hidden, non-wheezing variation)
- Hiccups
- No deep breathing, or hyperventilation
- Diaphragm, lung, or rib pain
- Swallowing air
- Reflux (GERD)
- Dental enamel erosion
- Ulcers
- Regurgitation, including dry heaves
- Waist Sensitivity
- Nausea
- Diminished, or excess, appetite
- Colic in infants, or children
- Diarrhea or Constipation
- Fatigue
- Hoarseness

- Coughing
- Pain: throat, chest, abdomen, shoulders, spine, extremities, back
- Arthritis
- Fatigue
- Nervousness, insecurity feelings
- Facial Flushing, blushing
- Depression
- Orthostatic hypotension
- Food, Chemical, Electromagnetic "Allergics"
- Pain in Neck or shoulder
- TMJ
- Bruxism
- Headaches
- Dizziness, poor balance
- Numbness, paralysis
- Hypoglycemia
- Shakiness, fainting
- Confusion
- Poor stress tolerance
- Vision weakness
- Pain anywhere can be made worse
- Learning/behavioral Problems
- Autism
- PMS
- Prostate problems
- Bladder weakness
- Obesity, or weight loss
- Intestinal Disease
- Gall Bladder Disease
- Adrenal Fatigue
- Hypothyroid, Hyperthyroid
- Kidney Disease
- Epilepsy
- Insomnia
- Sleep apnea—obstructive, or central
- Many Pregnancy Complaints
- Mast Cell Disease
- Porphyria—Acute Attacks

One key to an enlightened understanding of the VNI/HHS is that the amount of stomach protrusion is often irrelevant. In many people, serious illness begins unfolding even if the amount of protrusion is small. The Hiatal Hernia may be "small," for example on upper G.I. X-ray. In many sufferers, *any* such protrusion causes major hyper-excitability of the Vagus Nerve. Or—this researcher has found—*the Vagus Nerve may already be damaged/imbalanced from numerous, possible, underlying and hidden conditions.* These hidden, causative factors for the Vagus Nerve Imbalance must be tested and corrected (if possible) individually for wellness to be maintained. Allergies, heavy metal poisoning, parasitosis, porphyria, and other factors could *already* be imbalancing the Vagus Nerve.

The extensive Vagus Nerve is so diverse, and so interconnected to the visceral organs, that it has been nicknamed the "wanderer." The Vagus Nerve is the tenth cranial nerve, and is also called the pneumogastric nerve. It is the only nerve that starts in the brainstem—within the medulla—which contains the cardiac, respiratory, vomiting, and vasomotor centers, and involves autonomic functions, such as breathing, heart rate, blood pressure, maintaining consciousness, and regulating the sleep cycle. Figures 2 and 3 show that the Vagus Nerve innervates the crucial visceral organs (heart, lungs, gastrointestinal (GI) tract, pancreas, liver, kidneys, stomach), and also conveys sensory information about the state of these visceral organs, to the central nervous system (brain and spinal cord).

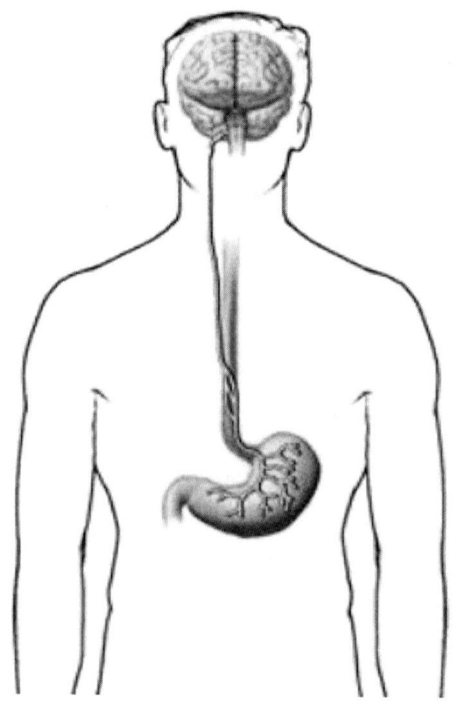

Figure 2. The Vagus Nerve innervating the stomach

The Vagus Nerve is part of the *Parasympathetic Nervous System* (adrenergic), which must be in balance with the Sympathetic Nervous System (cholinergic). Both are part of the Autonomic Nervous System, and are thus involved in cardiac muscle, and smooth muscle, regulation. Recently a third neurone system was found that works with the above two, but is regulated by nitric oxide, and primarily regulates the lungs and GI tract. Adrenergic means regulated by the hormones/neurotransmitters, epinephrine and norepinephrine; and cholinergic means regulated by the neurotransmitter, acetylcholine.

The slightest upward displacement of the stomach through the diaphragm disorders the Vagus Nerve, or worsens its *already* imbalanced nature, if that was the case. Immediately the stomach and *diaphragm* malfunction.

Over- or under-production of hydrochloric acid may result. Heart and lungs no longer function optimally. The entire digestive process also may then be adversely affected.

Figure 3. The Vagus Nerve's branches to the visceral organs. See also the back cover for the color version.

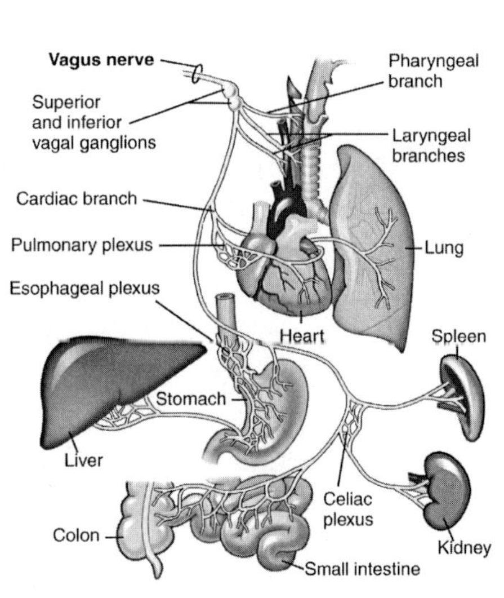

From an imbalanced Vagus Nerve, any other organ can begin to malfunction depending on genetic weaknesses, and various other factors. Of course, the diaphragm itself will directly be affected, and breathing normally no longer occurs. Other openings in the diaphragm—itself now stressed, stretched or torn— allow some major blood vessels to and from the heart to pass through it. Thus spasms in the abdominal aorta, and inferior vena cava can occur. The heart itself can be crowded, and pressed on, by the stomach being "where it doesn't belong." These factors, and the direct hyper-excitability of the Vagus Nerve's connection to the heart, lead to many Emergency Room visits and "pseudo-heart attack" symptoms of chest pain, difficulty breathing, and arm numbness.

The reader, if experiencing these complaints, should seek emergency medical care, and not assume they are arising from the HHS.

When French President Sarkozy collapsed in July, 2009, he spent the night in the hospital, and it was diagnosed as a Vagus Nerve problem.[4] The doctors said it was "minor." Translation into logic: If it had affected his heart a little bit more, and he then suffered a heart attack, it would no longer be "minor"—but would then not likely later be traceable back to his Vagus Nerve.

There is a remarkable similarity between the Hiatal Hernia Syndrome and angina. Both can cause similar symptoms, and both can occur after similar events such as overeating, exercise, and heavy lifting. My own hypothesis is that the Hiatal Hernia Syndrome, if uncorrected, may sometimes eventually lead to angina, and/or other heart conditions. Also I have noted that every person I have seen with either atrial fibrillation or supraventricular tachycardia (SVT) had hiatal hernia. It usually takes years before it gets to serious cardiac complaints, but dealing with the VNI/HHS, and also muscle trigger points[5] may be the best long-term solution if these are the ultimate causes of the heart rhythm disorders. Any degenerative heart condition may ultimately result from, or be exacerbated by, the VNI/HHS.

Pregnant women, for the obvious reason, need *frequent* Hiatal Hernia corrections—as do obese people, body builders and others whose exercise regimen, or type of work, stresses this area. The corrections below can provide remarkable relief for many complaints. Now the Hiatal Hernia can readily result from the trauma of birth. This will be undetected unless a good kinesiologist, or chiropractor, is around to perform surrogate muscle-testing on the infant. Now the end of this book will reveal that there is a possible link between Hiatal Hernia Syndrome and life expectancy. I would propose a long-term study, from birth, to learn statistically what illnesses correlate with Hiatal Hernia, as well as the Hiatal Hernia's possible use as a predictor of life expectancy.

Some kinesiologists, or chiropractors, will pull the stomach gently down on newborns possibly preventing a lifetime of illness. I initially use various trigger points, and not the "pull-down," which usually allows for the dropping of the stomach. I can also imagine that the Hiatal Hernia Syndrome could arise before birth from weeks or months of being somewhat "scrunched" in the womb. Physical trauma to the abdomen—at any time—can also cause a Hiatal Hernia. Even emotional stress can cause or exacerbate this condition.

The involvement of the HHS/VNI in emotional stress is illustrated with the following. A client flew in to see me. I balanced his HHS/VNI. I also did some phobia balancing on him. I saw that nothing lasted when he merely thought about being forced to take anti-hypertension medication. So I tested this, and tried to correct it. I saw that just thinking about the issue made his hernia reappear.

I then decided to hold down his stomach directly, after the last time I re-set these imbalances. I held down his upper stomach, and asked him to think again about taking those drugs, or even getting his blood pressure taken in the physician's office. Despite my trying to keep it down, as soon as he thought of the issue, I felt *his stomach scoot back up past my hands*. It truly had a mind of its own. For a moment, I thought of the scene in the movie, *Alien*, where the creature—previously hidden in John Hurt's abdomen—comes out and scoots past the others.

This client did not like being forced to take drugs, and so it was a deep issue for him, as he wanted to work on that problem in his own way. It shows though, how stress—even merely thinking of an issue—can make things more problematic.

There is a strong genetic component, as many family members have the Hiatal Hernia Syndrome, and often intestinal (umbilical) hernias and, in males, other hernias such as varicocele (testicular hernia.) There is a strong allergy connection to VNI/HHS. There's a vicious cycle between allergies and the HHS. Each one is capable of causing or exacerbating the other. In fact, I would like to note a possible, remarkable connection of a VNI/HHS symptom, and a well-known allergy test. This is the Coca Pulse test, which denotes an increase in pulse rate some time after eating a food (allergen). But one of the most common VNI/HHS symptoms is an increase in pulse rate! So I hypothesize that many food allergy sufferers, and their practitioners, who have used the Coca Pulse test for allergy detection, may also have been dealing (unbeknownst) with Hiatal Hernias.

To get well, one often has to learn to give up one's favorite foods as these are usually allergy/addictions. Once a Hiatal Hernia exists, it may worsen with every passing day, with every stress, and with every meal eaten (especially if it's an allergenic, or large, meal). Eventually this can result in very serious disease, unless uncovered and corrected, and unless the appropriate diet and lifestyle changes are made.

The Hiatal Hernia Syndrome may be the earliest cause of GERD (Gastroesophageal Reflux Disease), though the orthodox literature often only denotes "an occasional link." I believe many people have had Hiatal Hernia for some time, before GERD develops.

Helpful Recommendations for Hiatal Hernia Syndrome

- Eat small meals
- Chew food well—30 times
- Elevate the top of the bed by 6-9 inches, and/or get a wedge to sleep on
- Sleep on memory foam, after it outgasses—if you have MCS
- Don't eat spicy foods
- Lose weight, if possible
- Avoid alcohol, tobacco
- Avoid nightshades: tomato, potato, peppers
- Avoid or get muscle tested for dairy, wheat, vinegar, citrus
- Avoid fried or greasy foods, fats and *all* oils
- Avoid mints
- Avoid nuts, seeds, popcorn, or anything hard
- Avoid soda, seltzer
- Avoid tight clothing at the waist
- Don't eat less than 3 hours before going to sleep, unless porphyric, or hypoglycemic
- Try liquid diet, juicing, or baby food, if suffering greatly
- Avoid food that is too hot or too cold
- Don't eat too much roughage
- Be wary of taking too many tablets or capsules at once
- Master the Trigger Points, or "Pull down"

The above are things to do, not merely to read, if you wish to overcome this problem. Start now.

Bed elevation is crucial for the HHS. It may be a shock to learn, but *until about 150 years ago, many people slept in the seated position*—against a wall or such. Elevate the top of the bed 6-9 inches, by placing cinder blocks, or anything, under the front posts. And you can get a wedge to sleep on. You can do both. Some wedges even have memory foam on top. Get memory foam padding—either a new mattress, or the less expensive 2-4 inch overlay—for the whole bed to prevent, and to overcome, trigger points. The new padding may need to be outgassed for several weeks or months before use, for those with MCS (Multiple Chemical Sensitivities). Some sources recommend sleeping on the back or left side only. Avoid right side sleeping. If you have certain heart conditions, you may also have to avoid left side sleeping as well. Lifting, bending, sneezing, coughing, stress, and many other factors can immediately push the stomach (further?) up through the diaphragm.

Diet constraints cannot be overemphasized. Eating only small meals is crucial. Getting complete food allergy testing—via kinesiology is recommended here—and possibly rotating foods to avoid new food allergies can be crucial. Avoiding greasy and spicy foods is also essential. I have found that roughage may have disastrous consequences for the Hiatal Hernia Syndrome sufferer. The fiber may immediately push the stomach back up, or worsen the condition itself. Likewise for nuts and seeds. So only soft foods, cooked foods or juices should be allowed at first. Indeed I have made the following hypothesis.

A pure juice diet may have healing potential at least, in part, because the liquid diet may allow the VNI/HHS to heal! Likewise, I have surmised that taking supplements may cause or exacerbate the Hiatal Hernia Syndrome. The hard tablets and capsules, (until they dissolve), may also push the stomach right back up through the diaphragm. I have had clients say, "All supplements make me sick." Muscle testing on clients often reveals most clients are "allergic" to many of the supplements they take everyday, but never "all." So perhaps the client is just reporting how the supplements push the stomach back up. Some people take dozens of supplements *at the same time.* Not recommended! Pulling capsules apart, and putting the contents in a liquid, may be necessary, or else cut down on supplements, until healing has occurred.

Previously, as a general wellness modality, I recommended fasting. In theory, this might help heal this condition. However, due to possible hypothyroid, or porphyria conditions, I can no longer recommend fasting. Always remember that any food or supplement that shocks the stomach or esophagus can immediately bring back the Hiatal Hernia. Let us take an important detour now to the esophagus.

The Lower Esophageal Sphincter (LES), Schatzki's Ring & The Esophageal Longitudinal Muscle Contraction—A Cause of the HHS?

Some of the complaints attributable to the HH, may be caused by the so-called *Schatzki's ring,* and not the hernia itself—or by both. You can have one and not the other, or you may have both—as is common. Schatzki's ring is a disorder of the **Lower Esophageal Sphincter (LES)**. The LES acts like a valve between the esophagus, and the stomach. Schatzki's ring is a hardened, thickened, multi-fold, scar-type tissue. If this ring is present, the LES doesn't function properly. It may be open when it should be closed—causing reflux (GERD); or it may be closed when it should be open. The latter condition may trap food above the ring. There may be constriction. Trapped food, or spasms of the esophagus, can then cause breathing difficulty (asthma, etc.), tachycardia, or other arrhythmia. Schatzki's Ring should show up on upper GI X-ray, or endoscopy.

Breads, and fibrous (tough) meats are more likely to get trapped at the LES ring. Dry foods (like bread) can be a problem, but allergy may also be a factor. "Steakhouse Syndrome" is the nickname E.R. personnel have given this syndrome: people coming in with anxiety, respiratory, cardiac, or cardiac-like symptoms due to trapped food at the LES.

Any hard food, tablet or capsule can also get stuck. The person likely has some swallowing difficulties. Foods may need to be puréed in advanced cases; peristalsis may be impaired. In the E.R., sometimes an emergency endoscopy, and food or tablet removal is performed. Endoscopic *stretching* of the ring—via an inserted tool—may be recommended for Schatzki's Ring, *if there is esophageal narrowing*, and if the person has swallowing difficulty, or other complaints. Some people report improvement in their health after this. Some report that it only lasts six months to a year, and get it done every year.

The cause of Schatzki's Ring is "officially" unknown. O. Arthur Stiennon, M.D. hypothesized that the entire LES/HHS is caused by a *hypercontraction of the longitudinal muscle of the esophagus.*[6] Stiennon speculated that the Hiatal Hernia, LES Ring, and hypo-or hyperacidity/GERD/Reflux, and swallowing difficulties all stem from **Esophageal Longitudinal Muscle Contraction (ELMC)**. *This contraction then forcibly pulls up the stomach.* (One can test the esophagus kinesiologically, and put energy back into it with kinesiology, or reflexology.)

Stiennon speculated that the following factors might be causing this ELMC. These include *progesterone imbalance*—explaining possibly the frequency of hiatal hernia in pregnancy; and intestinal hormones—namely *CCK* and *secretin*. Fats entering the duodenum trigger CCK secretion, which is known to trigger smooth muscle contraction of the gallbladder, which then secretes bile into the duodenum.

The systemic release of CCK could cause or exacerbate the contraction of the esophageal longitudinal muscle, and the whole syndrome. Thus avoiding all fats, oils (including olive and flaxseed), meats, and dairy, may help alleviate this syndrome. So we see that the ELMC may itself be due to anomalies in the small intestine, and/or gallbladder. *A primarily, or exclusively, vegetarian diet may be needed, if the problem occurs from dietary fats/oils.* Stiennon noted that gallbladder (or bile problems) may be at the heart of this, as removing it stops heartburn in some people. (I assert that hidden porphyrics do not tolerate supplements that increase bile.)

Stiennon says that *H. pylori* in the duodenum may be a causative factor. (I would add the possibility of other microorganism overgrowths as well.) He also states that Barrett's Esophagus is *not* a cancerous, or pre-cancerous, condition, rather it is another aspect of a hyper-contracted ELMC, accompanied by reflux. Recently, deficiency of Vasoactive Intestinal Polypeptide (VIP) has been found in people with chronic and/or "allergic" illnesses. And the VIP hormone has widespread function in the body. It affects the pancreas, heart (possible CHF factor), and the brain's sleep center. It is known to relax the LES, stomach, and gallbladder. Could this deficiency be one of the causes of the HHS/VNI?

I think trigger points (muscle knots) could cause the ELMC, as they are deeply entwined with muscle spasm. The Vagus Nerve is likely involved in the beginning, or at the end of this syndrome, or both. Scars can cause trigger points. Tonsillectomy, and resultant throat scar, can be causative here. Of course, the reason the person may have "needed" a tonsillectomy is that throat problems already existed. Any allergic reaction to any food may play a role. The throat itself may start a chain reaction. Some people have an excess of "complement"—an immune system component—in their throats. An adverse reaction could start with chewing/swallowing a reacting food. Then the Vagus Nerve goes hyper, and the longitudinal muscles of the esophagus spasm, and pull the stomach up—and on the scenario goes. I have seen chicken and/or its fat do this with several people.

Getting back to the Hiatal Hernia now, avoiding caffeine, and any other neurotoxins, and/or excitotoxins, such as the ubiquitous MSG, (Monosodium Glutamate), or aspartame is important. Perhaps the most nerve-damaging substance is mercury. Perhaps too the Vagus Nerve, due to its high metabolic rate, preferentially absorbs mercury, or other toxins, more than other nerve tissue? And this combination of VNI/HHS and mercury can be devastating. The Vagus Nerve, like the hernia itself, probably needs time to heal, and for everything to be done right for a span of several months, or it may have been permanently damaged by toxins. Soda—with the extra gas it contains—should be avoided.

Trapped gas makes this syndrome much worse. Indeed the sufferer may have episodes of feeling as if dying, sometimes accompanied by a racing heart, hypertension, and asthma—or some breathing difficulty—only to be relieved by belching, or perhaps the gas passes down the other way unnoticeably.

Proper food combining may help prevent gas. Avoid protein and carbs at the same meal. When the stomach goes back down, much gurgling is often audible. One hundred years ago, medical schools taught Roemheld's (or Gastro-Cardiac) Syndrome which described significant cardiac complaints arising from stomach problems. Unfortunately, this now seems to have disappeared from all but the homeopathic, medical literature. Similarly, ancient medical literature described asthma as a *stomach-originating complaint.*

Medical testing for the Hiatal Hernia may miss it. Less expensive is the Upper GI X-ray series, done after ingesting a radioactive "milkshake." To help find the Hiatal Hernia—after missing many—some tilting of the patient was added during the procedure. The far more involved test is the endoscopy (EGD). This may sometimes miss the HHS also—if the anesthetic/sedative relaxes the system sufficiently—and the stomach temporarily drops out of the diaphragm.

Some gastroenterologists use a numbing, throat spray at the outset. Others have found this is often allergenic, and unnecessary. The video camera that the endoscopic tube contains, reveals the status of esophageal, gastric and duodenal tissues.

Ulcerations, inflammations, and growths are looked for. The tube/device is also used to take biopsies. These tissues are then tested for cancer or pre-cancerous conditions and to look for bacteria, especially the ulcer-causing *Helicobactor pylori*. This examination also looks for the allegedly, pre-cancerous, esophageal condition called Barrett's Esophagus, which can occur after long-term GERD. The Hiatal Hernia *may* be found with either the upper GI X-rays, or the endoscopy.

It may not be possible to completely overcome the VNI/HHS unless the sufferer becomes thin. This can be difficult due to other conditions. Many forms of exercise will exacerbate the hernia. Finding some exercise regimen that doesn't worsen the hernia is important, as is taking it slow and steady. It may be very problematic to become thin as one complaint for the VNI/HHS is that eating when the stomach is up may immediately cause the sufferer to get *hungrier* (and not satiated) as s/he eats! Over-eating—one of the worst things for this condition—often results, along with obesity.

Hypoglycemia may be caused by this condition. But sometimes glucose testing, when these assumed hunger pains arise, reveals that no standard, simple low blood sugar disease exists. But there are other more complicated illnesses that many practitioners do not know about—but you do now. Stomach hyper-acidity often masquerades as "hypoglycemia" feelings as well.

I suspect many cases of "hypoglycemia" may either really be the VNI/HHS, and not hypoglycemia, or at least that the VNI/HHS is one of the exacerbating factors of hypoglycemia—as well as are allergies, parasitosis, and porphyria. I was astounded once myself when I was feeling "out of it." My glucose meter revealed a blood sugar of only 60, which is low, and low for me. I had one of my students test me for Hiatal Hernia. My stomach was up, and I showed him what to do to get my stomach to drop below the diaphragm. I felt that "assumed low blood sugar feeling" immediately go away. I was amazed to see the glucose meter then read 90!

The VNI/HHS can be one of the great, hidden causes of obesity. However, when the Vagus Nerve is perhaps even more imbalanced, *a loss of appetite* may result. The sufferer is then in an even more dangerous condition, perhaps with significant, adrenal failure at that point.

The HHS/VNI commonly causes phobias, panic attacks, or anxiety. The sufferer must become his/her own expert. Simple energy testing for the HH is in the next section. In general, energy testing and balancing is often a crucial, neglected aspect of a symptom or condition; but it is not a substitute for medical testing and evaluation.

The illnesses of children need special mention. There has been an epidemic of asthma, dyslexia, learning and behavioral problems in children during the last several decades. Once again, I assert that VNI/HHS is a large part of the cause of these illnesses in children, and of the asthma epidemic (in both adults and children). Asthma—often a non-wheezing, *undiagnosed* variation that includes locked-up chest muscles—may be one of the most frequent "side effects" of the Hiatal Hernia. It is never "too early" to get the stomach down. I have found children with learning and behavioral disorders such as dyslexia, ADD, ADHD, Aspergers Syndrome, autism, asthma and allergies, almost always have the VNI/HHS.

The hyperactive child's inability to "sit still" could actually occur because the *seated position* often makes the VNI/HHS much worse! Most seats may be very unnatural and may further stress the hernia. (If my stomach is up, I sometimes eat standing up. And my car's seat can aggravate my Hiatal Hernia.) Getting back to children. As stated earlier, there is often a terrible synergism between mercury toxicity, and VNI/HHS. The child, who suffers from these illnesses cited, often also has mercury poisoning as determined by Hair Mineral Analysis (which can easily be verified by blood mercury testing.) The child's mercury poisoning could have come from the preservative used in vaccinations (ethyl mercury, AKA thimerosal, a potent neurotoxin), or from leeching of the mother's dental amalgam when the child was a fetus; or from fish, or environmental sources. Mercury often induces hidden porphyria.

The parent can be taught how to get the child's stomach down. Mercury poisoning in particular, I have found, makes it difficult for the stomach to stay down. Unless and until mercury, and/or other toxins present, are eliminated, the stomach may not stay down. For this work to last, we also need complete and accurate testing for overgrowths of all "Critters" (Candida[7], protozoan parasites, viruses, bacteria—including *Helicobactor pylori*, and *Clostridium difficile*) that may be overgrowing in the body, including in the stomach. All overgrowths need to be eliminated.

There may be an intimate, even causal, relationship between hiatal hernia and asthma and possibly other respiratory disorders. For example, some researchers have noted a frequent occurrence of both GERD (reflux), and asthma, in children and adults. Some researchers believe that GERD may cause or influence asthma, and others say it's vice versa. Some physicians or researchers have found that treating either GERD, or asthma, sometimes helps the other condition when both occur in the same individual. I think that the earliest link and possible iniator of *both* may be the Hiatal Hernia.

Now in an informal study, I noted that an apparently large percentage of people with various respiratory diseases (including asthma, emphysema, bronchitis, COPD) either are aware that they also have a hiatal hernia (via an official diagnosis), or are being treated for GERD or heartburn, which I assert is nearly always a result, or an indicator, of the presence of hiatal hernia.

What I also propose is that *all* sufferers of respiratory disease who possess a known or "hidden" hiatal hernia may benefit significantly if they or their practitioners learn to get the stomach down and below the diaphragm—and more importantly and more problematically, try to keep it that way—regardless of the etiology. Sadly, this connection and method is not known to pulmonolgists, or respiratory therapists. The Hiatal Hernia continues to be thought of as an incidental condition, unrelated to anything!

I believe that the HHS is often the cause for the creation, or re-creation, of numerous trigger points. In particular, I found a deep connection of the HHS/VNI with respiratory and coronary Trigger Points later depicted in this book. And so neural therapy, or manual trigger point therapy, will be short lived unless, and until, the HHS/VNI is brought under control. In addition, porphyria, or fat intolerance, may be the cause of *both* 1. Why the stomach "doesn't stay down" and 2. Why the Vagus Nerve may be damaged even without having a Hiatal Hernia. We need to be individually tested for many factors to find the cause of our HHS/VNI.

Alleviating the Hiatal Hernia has (in some people) helped with all of the complaints or maladies listed at the start of this chapter. The HHS/VNI is either a primary cause, or an exacerbating factor, in these symptoms or illnesses. Some of these symptoms, or organ disorders, can arise from direct over-energy from the Vagus Nerve's connection to these organs, or by secondary nerve imbalance, as these other nerves interact with the Vagus Nerve, or from digestive disorder begun in the stomach, or by systemic pH imbalance. Of course, when we don't breathe right, oriental knowledge has revealed that any imbalance can then result. Then there is the possibly related matter of hypocapnia—low CO_2 (carbon dioxide) level.

Likewise when adrenal exhaustion sets in, from the continual stress of the VNI/HHS, all the other organs in the body will weaken. Fixing, or attempting to fix, *resultant* problems is of very limited value, unless and *until the earliest causative factors are found and dealt with*, if possible. And the reason the Hiatal Hernia Syndrome is considered to be "minor" by the medical orthodoxy, is because most of medicine has not observed how so many seemingly, unconnected illnesses can often be immediately improved by getting the stomach below the diaphragm. Of course, decades—perhaps a lifetime—usually goes by without most people ever getting their "hidden" Hiatal Hernias corrected. The illnesses it has (directly or indirectly) caused will then be even harder to connect to the VNI/HHS.

I would urge anyone with any of these problems to add this to his/her protocol of things to do. As I stated above, over 90% of people I have seen with severe food, chemical, or electromagnetic sensitivities have the VNI/HHS as one causative factor in their sensitivities. This can be a very tricky thing to uncover oneself. E.g., many clients have said the following to me: "I can't figure out what I am allergic to!" Now sometimes this may be said by someone who is not taking responsibility, and/or is in an addictive state.

But this may not always be the case; and I note the following. (Even a food diary may not help if the following scenario is in play.) Let's say someone eats something and does not react to it as s/he eats this food, when the stomach is down (VNI/HHS in balance), so there is no reaction. Then a few days later, the person first eats some lettuce at night, or takes twenty vitamin pills. The fiber, or the pills, before the person goes to sleep, causes the stomach to move up (through the diaphragm), or some other stress does this.

The next morning when the subject eats the food that did not provoke an "allergic" or sensitivity reaction the last time, s/he now suffers a reaction. Or possibly any food will make the Hiatal Hernia sufferer "react" at that point in time. Because of Vagus Nerve Imbalance and/or stomach imbalance, the gastrointestinal tract may now be in a hyper-reactive state, and that undigested food will now get into the blood stream. From there it can directly shock any organ, or possibly provoke an antibody-antigen reaction.

So we see the intimate relationship between the VNI/HHS, and food sensitivities. *But a hyper-excited Vagus Nerve will make the subject over-reactive to any change in his/her environment, including chemical substances, and electromagnetic fields.* This is further magnified by the subject having weak adrenals and/or thyroid glands, which are needed to counter any stress. Summing up, the VNI/HHS can cause or exacerbate allergies, and vice-versa.

In some people, the *intermittent* nature of their symptoms, and allergy-like reactions to foods, chemicals and EMF, is related to the aptly named Acute *Intermittent* Porphyria (AIP). When their *hidden* porphyria is in an elevated state, the Vagus Nerve is more out of balance, and they will be sicker, more anxiety-ridden, and suffering from allergy-like reactions to foods, chemicals, EMF, or all of them, as well *as more intolerant of emotional stress, environmental temperature, light, sound, and any stimulus.* All the defects in the body are revealing themselves at the same time because of overarching imbalances in play, including the many organs connected to the Vagus Nerve, hypocapnia, hyponatremia, porphyrin toxicity, or other generalized imbalances.

Another factor that may relate to the Vagus Nerve is its diurnal cycle (high/low during 24 hours). Are you sicker, and more "allergic" to foods, chemicals, or EMF at certain times of the day? If you know you have porphyria, are you more likely to have acute attacks in the early morning, or late at night? This variation in your health, energy level, reactivity, etc., may be related to variations in your Vagus Nerve's energy level (diurnal cycle) throughout the day. It could also be related to adrenal hormone variation, or other factor. And all these could be inter-related. But make use of this knowledge to either try to fix/balance things when they are at their weakest, and/or to avoid any stressors—including foods, chemicals, EMF, etc.—when you are at your weakest.

MCS sufferers who are used to blaming the chemicals "out there" for all problems need to learn that when the Vagus Nerve is imbalanced, may be the time when he/she will be most likely to over-react to chemicals! It may be that: "as your Vagus Nerve goes, so goes your allergies/sensitivities." Of course, I am not in favor of the prevalence of these toxic, environmental chemicals, or EMF. But the sufferers of these allergy-like reactions must find out what is different about the *inside* of their bodies, in order to get better, and to prevent a worsening of their problems. The VNI/HHS, and any factors that may be causing or exacerbating it, may be a crucial in elucidating the nature of chronic allergies, chronic fatigue, and chronic, degenerative illness.

Before hopefully getting the stomach down/out of the diaphragm, various techniques may be needed to correct an imbalanced or misshapen diaphragm. This then normalizes the diaphragm's movement. The longer one has had this undiagnosed, untreated HHS/VNI, the more likely it is that one has a "stuck diaphragm." It is also most likely to exist if there is chest pain, rib pain, and trouble breathing, and bloating.

The diaphragm is controlled by the **Phrenic Nerve** (see Fig. 15), which does interact with the Vagus Nerve. Those performing either needle or electric acupuncture have actually had success with respiratory collapse by working on the LI17 (Large Intestine 17) point. This is the point that relates to the Phrenic Nerve. It's in the neck region, and is also near the carotid artery and the larynx—and can be precarious to work on. So it is beyond the scope here. In one study—that connected needles to an electrical stimulating device—it was reported that, "Eighty-two comatose patients without spontaneous respiration were treated [on the LI17point.] *Respiration resumed in all cases.*"[8] (Italics added here.) One case involved "chemical poisoning." The electrical stimulation was a sawtooth wave with a frequency ranging from 16-25/min., which is close to the human respiration frequency, and is thus known as a respiratory wave. I also occasionally use the SCENAR (electrical) device, in conjunction with my advanced kinesiology methods.

We are ready now to proceed to restore balance to the Vagus Nerve, diaphragm and the stomach.

Section II

Corrections For

The Hiatal Hernia

and

Vagus Nerve Imbalance

and the Diaphragm

Corrections For The Hiatal Hernia and Vagus Nerve Imbalance

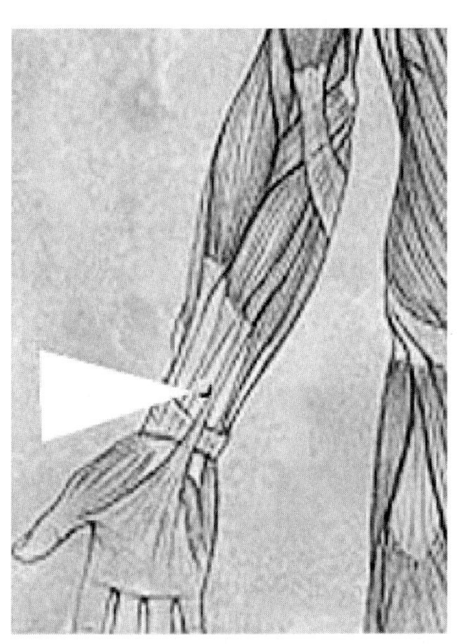

Let's start to make things better!

Figure 4—Vagus Nerve Point Tapping. Tap the PC 6 point 30 times, both sides.

The first correction to help the HHS/VNI is to **calm the Vagus Nerve.** We restore balance to the Vagus Nerve by tapping the PC 6 (Pericardium 6) acupuncture point; it relates to the Vagus Nerve. See Fig. 4. Tap—with the tips of your middle and pointer fingers—both arm points 30 times. The point is 2 "cun" below the wrist crease. (A Chinese cun is your own thumb width, at its joint.) You can even tap with a waltz beat—Hard-soft-soft. This can relax the Vagus Nerve. So can lightly holding—for up to several minutes—points on the forehead as depicted in Fig. 10. Note that if the corrections in this book do not last long, it may mean there are other problems ongoing. In (usually) hidden porphyrics, the Vagus Nerve, in some cases, has even been found to be partially demyclimated. [See my *Porphyria* book for more on this.] Ice can also be held on the PC 6 point.

Corrections for the diaphragm can include rubbing or stretching certain body points, or working on the diaphragm itself. The abdominal aorta and inferior vena cava may suffer fewer spasms when the diaphragm is corrected. See Figure 5 for this.

Figure 5. Diaphragm correction.

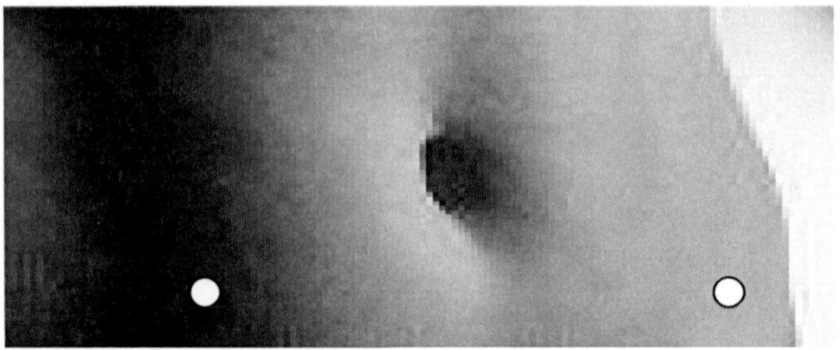

Re-set the diaphragm by rubbing hard the two points (white dots) shown in Figure 5, for 10-20 seconds. These are (for an average adult) two inches to each side of the navel, and one inch below it. *Don't hold your breath during any correction.*

Fig 6. Coronary Trigger Points: Adjacent to the Sternum, at the level of 3, 4, and 5 ribs. Or anywhere in the Pectoralis muscles.

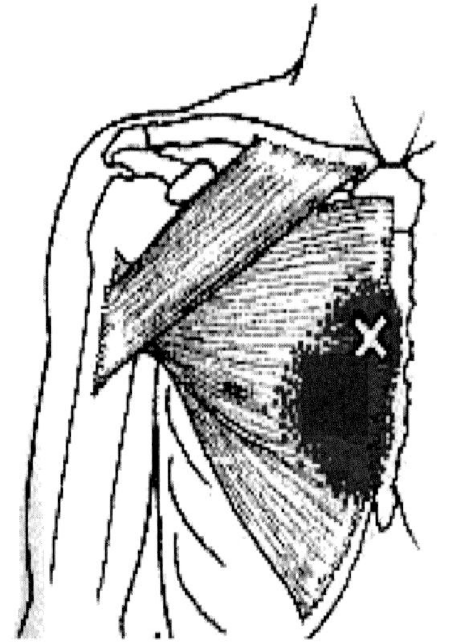

Instead of rushing to try to "pull the stomach down," which often aggravates the problem in some people, I try to re-set certain crucial trigger points, which often allow the stomach to drop down on its own. The first set of points we use are **the Philibert Coronary Reflex Trigger Points**[9]: See Fig. 6. These are *between the ribs* at their junction with the sternum, at the levels of the 3rd-5th ribs—the so-called intercostals (the "X" in Fig. 6 is one of the six points)—on both sides, of the sternum. That's two sets (both sides) of three points—or **a total of six points.** I would add that any painful spot(s), or muscle knots, *anywhere* in the "pecs"/breast muscles should also be worked on, especially if there is also any heart or lung problem. Manual treatment of the

Coronary Trigger Points involves pressing into them for at least 10 seconds each. These points can relax the heart and coronary arteries, acording to Dr. Philibert. The more a trigger point hurts when worked on, the more it is said, you will benefit—provided there isn't any damage at these points. Do not work on vulnerable areas such as the spinal vertebrae.

Figure 7. Infraspinatus Trigger Points

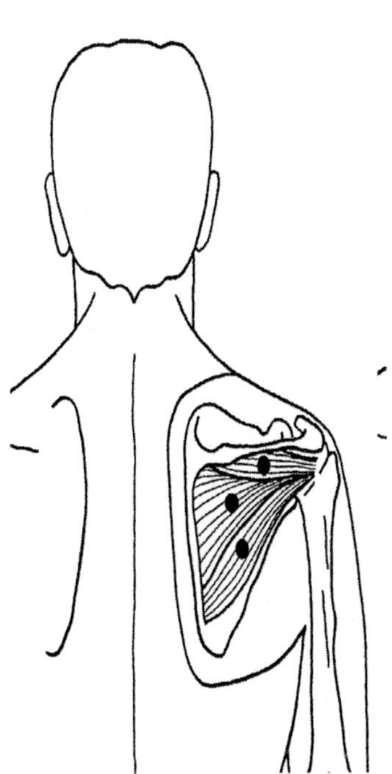

Sometimes the above correction also allows the stomach to drop down below the diaphragm, thus halting the whole HHS/VNI affair, at least temporarilly. But sometimes, the Respiratory Reflex points are needed as well, or instead. These points can relax your breathing apparatus, according to Dr. Philibert. And re-seting them may allow your stomach to drop down on its own, I have found.

The **Philibert Infraspinatus Respiratory Reflex Trigger Points.** See Figure 7. Fixing this set of trigger points can truly relax your breathing. Doing this can be a great and immediate help for asthmatics, and for sufferers of other respiratory problems. If present, you will find a taut band of muscle on the back of the shoulder blade (on either, or both sides). This often is very near the SI 11 acupunture point—*middle point* in the drawing above, right. (SI refers to Small Intestine.) You will need either a partner to rub the point, or buy a curved body tool that you can then use to apply pressure yourself to points on your back. Now you should find the actual taut band(s) of muscle. When you, (or your partner) have found a taut band of muscle in the SI 11 region, or *anywhere* on the back of the shoulder blade, follow the general Bonnie Prudden methods[10] of trying to work it out. The trigger point is usually in the center of the taut band of muscle. First press hard into it for about 10 seconds. Then continue to press into it, while simultaneously pushing into at least the four directions of a compass (N, S, E, W), again for 10 seconds each time. Do both sides. Breathing should be more relaxed.

Hiatal Hernia Correction

If you feel that your stomach is down, you can stop, or proceed to relax the actual hernia area and help bring it down. If you know muscle testing, you can touch, and muscle test, the white dot, in Fig. 8, the Hiatal Hernia Test Point, which is 1" below the xiphoid process—which is in the center, where the ribs come together. The correction is to push a bit into the white dot with both thumbs, and then continue doing this as you move your thumbs down and to the left 4-6 inches, as the arrow shows. Breathe out as you do this. Some call this the "pull-down." You may also hold your fingers in at their final position, for a minute or longer. Some say this may make the correction last longer.

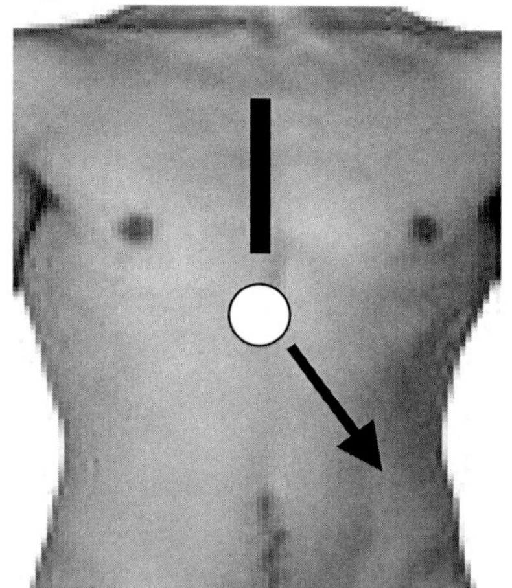

Figure 8. Hiatal Hernia Correction, (and also illustrated is part of the sternum/diaphragm correction.)

If starting this correction makes you feel worse, stop. If not, do it at least twice. Rest and see how you feel. You can do this several times per day. Before eating, and before sleeping, are good times to re-set your Hiatal Hernia. Do it very gently (at least at first), don't over-do it. Don't do it if you have much trapped gas. Don't do it if you think you might have some serious medical condition, like appendicitis, or any abdominal, medical problem. Rather seek medical attention if that is the case.

Additional, Related Hiatal Hernia Correction Options— Third Edition

1. Hold the diaphragm in place with one hand (pushing up and into it *gently—under the rib cage),* while pulling down the hernia, with the other hand. This is to prevent what may be happening much of the time. Just pulling down without this addition may further stress and move the diaphragm.

2. Instead of pulling in the diagonal direction, as in Figure 8, going straight down some 3-6 inches or so, may sometimes be preferable.

3. Once you have pushed down—either diagonally or straight down—*hold it there for a while.* Ease up after a while. The interval could be up to several minutes.

4. The need for the above methods is best gauged by the advanced method we teach, of asking the body questions, and getting it to assay the situation and, via muscle testing (Applied Kinesiology) to tell the testor, which option(s) should be used.

5. Instead of any pulling down, the most advanced method is to "lock the problem" in, and ask the body what methods it gauges would help at the time. Any thing from: supplements to energy balancing, and many more possibilities, could come up during this advanced method. Our brains record every imbalance in the body, and

> know—if asked in a certain way—the optimal way to correct it.
>
> 6. If things still do not last, it may be the body's way of saying there are other, serious underlying problems present that must be addressed. These can include, porphyria, mast cell disease, cardiac problems, etc.

Sometimes, after the stomach goes down, the subject smiles and feels like they are breathing right for the first time in many years. The subject often reports standing taller, and feeling stronger, than s/he has in a while! I have seen oxygen saturation go from 88% to 98%, after Hiatal Hernia correction. I have also seen body temperature go up several degrees to the norm of 98.6. F. I have also seen blood sugar levels go from a hypoglycemic 60 to a normal 90, immediately after HH correction.

Sometimes, however, there is discomfort in the abdomen. The person feels really bad. This may be due to a skin factor. If it is the skin factor, I can almost always fix this with a skin proprioceptor correcting technique. The actual technique is to pull, stretch and vibrate the skin.

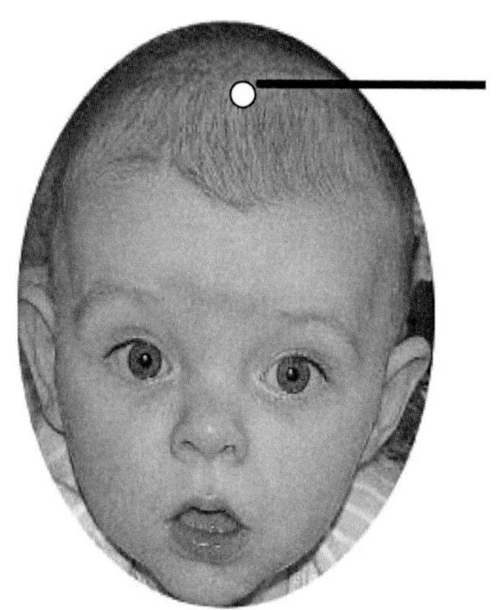

Figure 9. The Anterior Fontanel, or "baby's soft spot."

You can **hold the Anterior Fontanel point (Figure 9) lightly, while rubbing the sternum (Figure 8) for 20 seconds to further balance the diaphragm**.

The Hiatal Hernia Syndrome sufferer's skin proprioceptors have likely been in a bad state for many years too. These can be supersensitive to touch, let alone a deep stretching. This is an indication, as well, of how the Vagus Nerve is likely also to be in a very bad, (hyper-excited), state. Remember, on some people, you cannot jump in and do the "pull down." It will worsen their already high anxiety feelings.

Now you can do some more techniques for your diaphragm. The bold line in Fig. 8, in the center, is the sternum. You can rub it hard while you gently hold the anterior fontanel, or "baby's soft spot" in Figure 9. This further helps relax or re-set your diaphragm.

Assuming I have tested for many other imbalances first, I then re-check them. It is indeed amazing to, (usually but not always), see blood sugar imbalance, thyroid, adrenal, small and/or large intestine, gallbladder, brain integration, pitch/roll/yaw (spatial imbalance), TMJ (sometimes though the TMJ can actually help fix the HHS), and many other "energy circuits" re-test as intrinsically fixed by the HHS correction. Of course, none of this is a substitute for proper medical testing, and treatment, for any of these problems. This refers to energy states only. Then comes the perennial question, "how long will it last?"

It may be difficult for some to keep the stomach down, and/or the Vagus Nerve balanced, due to factors already cited in this book. So, as with much of chronic illness, it is up to the sufferer to learn and master these factors, or get extra help if needed. But these diet and lifestyle changes can be mastered by all.

Additional energy balancing techniques from Applied Kinesiology can help calm the brain and/or stomach. These techniques can *get more blood flowing to the higher centers of the brain, stomach, and heart.* They are called neurovascular corrections, and they require a light touch. The first one—the **Anerior Fontanel** or "baby's soft spot"—is shown in Figure 9. You can hold it along with the two points in Fig. 10, the **Frontal Eminence** points, for 30 seconds to five minutes.

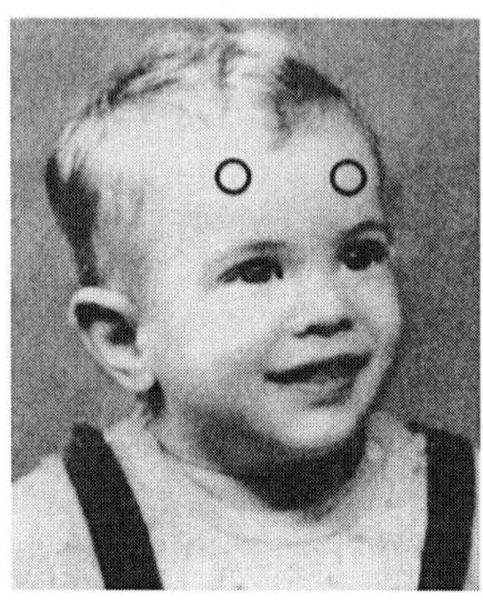

Figure 10. Frontal Eminence Points. (The author, circa age 2, before the dots were surgically removed.)

This points can balance the brain, and stomach. The frontal eminence points are also known as the **Emotional Stress Release** points. They are about 1 to 1.5 inches above the eyebrows, at the same level. Hold lightly 30 seconds to five minutes.

Reflexology for the solar plexus, diaphragm, pyloric valve, brain, esophagus, and other organs, can also help. See Figure 11. Press deeply and maintain for 10 seconds, at each point you are working on. Note the white dots for the Solar Plexus—within the diaphragm band. Separately apply deep, steady pressure to both regions, for 10-30 seconds. You should feel much better, as this "hypochondriacal" region gets balanced! (The ancients knew that discomfort in this region was real, and significant; and not "mental".) The brain points, on the big toes, will also help sufferers of CFS, porphyria, MCS, allergies, etc.

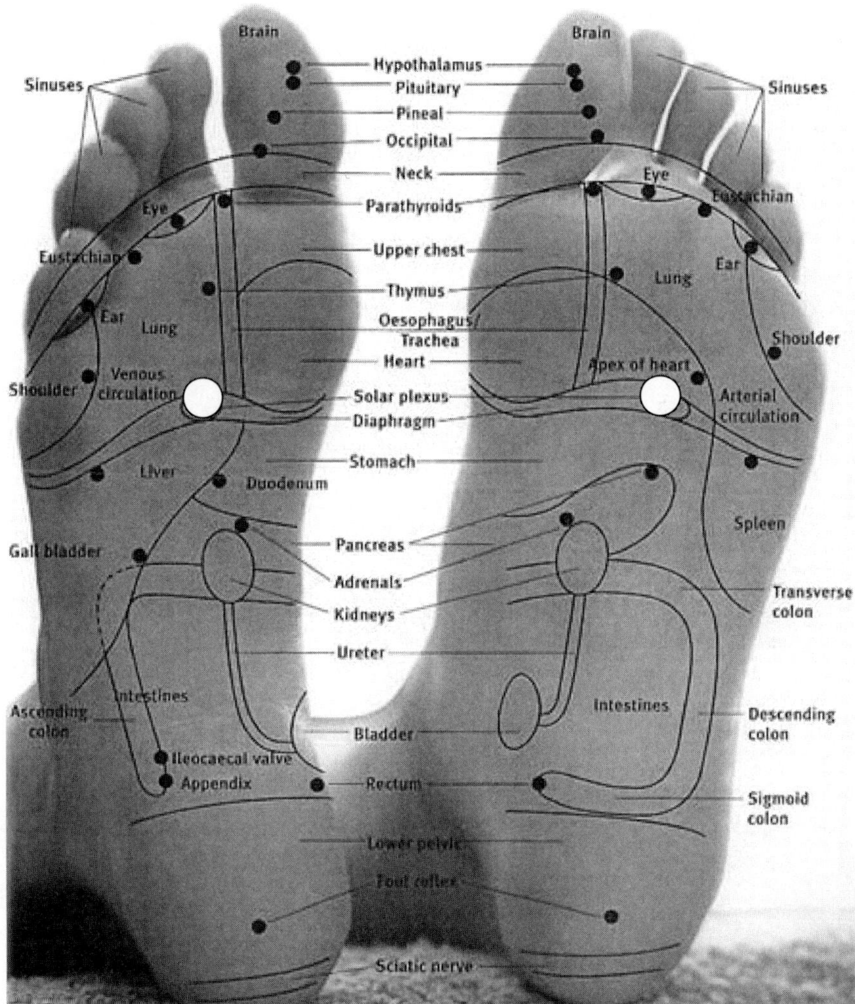

Figure 11. Foot reflexology.

Meditation techniques can also help keep you and your stomach stay in better balance. Ginger can help with stomach complaints, but muscle testing needs to first be done for the ginger, as you can react to its strong flavor. Everything must be done individually! You can also become allergic to something after taking it every day. Learning and practicing proper breathing methods can be a big help. The HHS/VNI may be a leading cause of hypocapnia, and possibly vice versa. The amino acid/neurotransmitter, GABA, or PharmaGABA may also help. Liposomal glutathione may help too, often before bedtime. Charcoal may help to adsorb gas—and even excess fats.

Fig. 12. Points & regions for placing foods, vitamins. for allergy testing. **Fig. 13. Basic Muscle testing** on an Aussie Rose. **Fig. 14. Basic testing**. Depictions from *Allergies & Candida* by the author. There is vastly more to having accurate muscle testing.

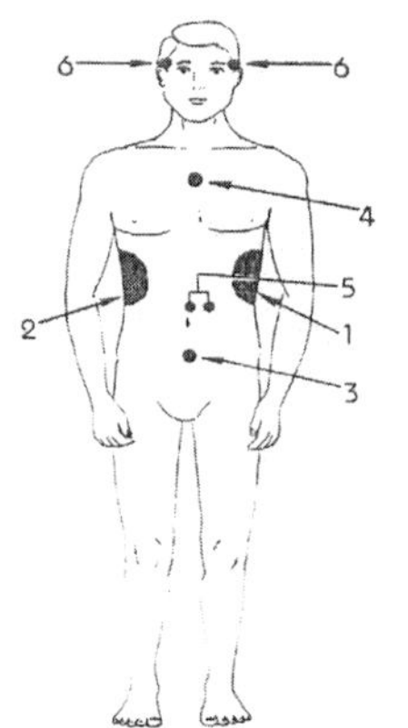
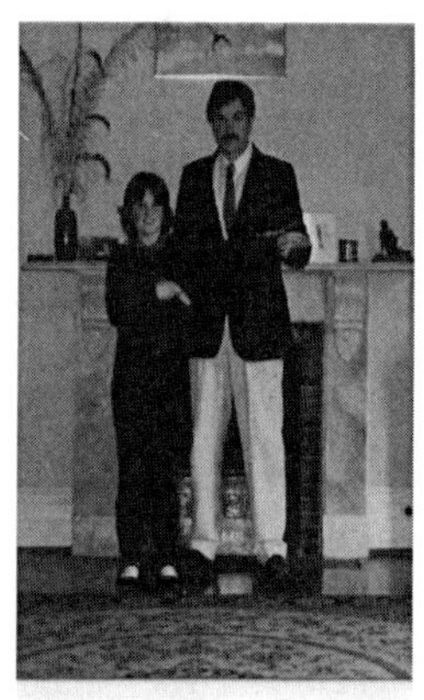
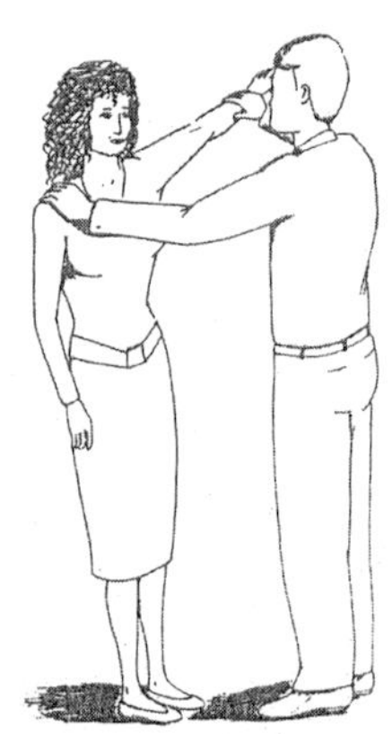

Beside ginger, the following herbal substances *may* help the HHS: comfrey, pepsin, aloe vera, Pau D'Arco, celery, and Swedish bitters. Useful homeopathic remedies include lycopodium, nux vomica, nux moschata, and others. These must all be muscle tested first. I trust the reader will realize that no neutraceutical is a substitute for keeping the stomach down, and for making the diet and lifestyle changes needed. Figures 12-14 depict allergy testing regions to place foods, and the basic muscle testing procedure. (There is much more to this.)

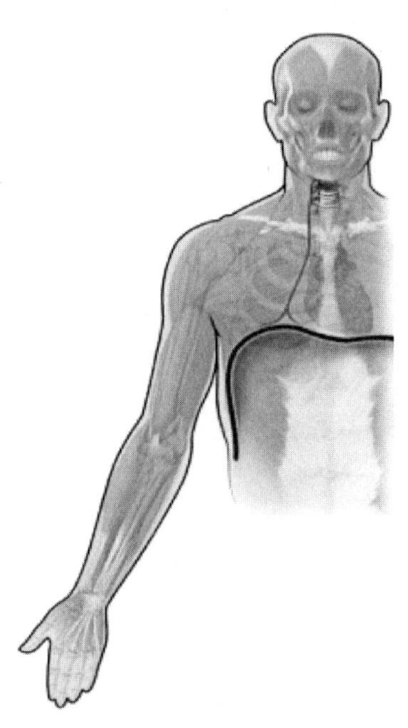

Figure 15. Phrenic Nerve—innervating the diaphragm. The Large Intestine 17 point, or Phrenic Nerve point—which is capable of restarting respiration, when appropriately stimulated—is in the neck region, about an inch above the collar bone.

Swallowing Difficulty Help

Before swallowing any solid or liquid, first *place your chin on, or toward, your chest.* Vagus Nerve Point tapping can also help.

Breathing Techniques[11] To Help Minor Heart or Lung Complaints, Anxiety, and other Problems

People with HHS/VNI find out that they have the syndrome usually by experiencing heart or respiratory symptoms; and medical testing reveals "no [other] serious organ disease exists." There are two breathing methods that can yield immediate and long-term relief here. They can be *crucial* to improving your HHS/VNI, and possibly many other health problems.

1. **Practice long, slow, deep exhalations.** Try to make your *lower* abdomen move properly as well. It comes up as you breathe in, and goes down into the body as you breathe out. Reverse breathing often exists in those with a stuck diaphragm. *Breathe out to a count at least twice as long as you breathe in to. Or try to see how long you can take to slowly breathe out. You can also purse your lips during the slow exhalations.*

2. What is now called the Buteyko method is **to practice intervals of shallow breathing and breath-holding** *to raise the regulating CO_2 blood level.* Also try to keep your **mouth closed** when having an attack, as the opposite tends to cause a reflex leading to more CO_2 loss.

People also ask about surgery. One gastroenterologist, I knew, advised against it as it often does not correct the problem, and can cause new ones. It wraps the upper third of the stomach around the esophagus. It does *not* pull the stomach down, and sew up the hole in the diaphragm, as one might think. You will not be able to throw up afterwards, even if you need to. First speak to people (physicians, and patients who have had it) other than the surgeon. If diet and lifestyle changes aren't made, it may not help. If they are made, it may not be needed. But the size of the hernia may be a factor.

To summarize, the Hiatal Hernia may be a frequent, undetected occurrence often from the trauma of birth, or from some stress or trauma thereafter. The Vagus Nerve is then immediately imbalanced. However, the Vagus Nerve may be imbalanced due to crucial, but hidden, problems cited in this book; and these factors must be tested individually. Through the mechanisms outlined here, virtually any organ can then be adversely affected.

For many people the amount of imbalance in the Vagus Nerve is the key. The VNI then allows any visceral organ to malfunction.

VNI also predisposes to trigger point creation, I hypothesize, and pain anywhere in the body. Corrections in this book for the VNI, diaphragm and the hiatal hernia can last as long as many months, or as brief as seconds. When the corrections are short-lived, it may mean that the diet and lifestyle corrections were not made, and/or that other medical problems exist. As cited earlier, these can include the PFO or other heart defect, hidden porphyria, mast call disease, or other factors. *The corrections should then be performed frequently, while the other factors are read up on and investigated and dealt with if found.*

So the VNI/HHS may be a primary cause of much chronic, degenerative physical and "mental" illness." The VNI/HHS may also be a cause of food, chemical and electromagnetic sensitivities. The Hiatal Hernia/Vagus Nerve Imbalance is a crucial syndrome that can eventually cause many other illnesses including heart and lung problems. I suggest the Hiatal Hernia may be a predictor of life expectancy.

A recent advance in cardiology is the sub-field of Heart Rate Variability (HRV).[12] HRV refers to statistical analyses of five-minute, (or longer), electrocardiograms. HRV analyses and subject follow-up for "all-cause mortality"[13] yielded the conclusion that *Heart Rate Variability is perhaps the best predictor of life expectancy.* But Heart Rate Variability and even stress, "stress vulnerability," and "reactivity to stress" have been demonstrated to be highly dependent on the state of the Vagus Nerve.

Thus we have come full circle and verified Carey Reams quote cited at the beginning of this book. Reams stated that illness began with problems with the Vagus Nerve. HRV studies have now found that *our life expectancies may depend on an optimum, or balanced Vagus Nerve; and the Vagus Nerve cannot be in balance, unless the stomach is down and stays down.*

Conclusion

The logical conclusion I propose here is that the Hiatal Hernia—overlooked, in its totality, by most of mainstream and alternative medicine—may indirectly be a great predictor of life expectancy! I first proposed this in 2002. Though this may be the first time this Hiatal Hernia/Longevity hypothesis has been explicitly stated, it should not come as a surprise. Since this problem—the Hiatal Hernia Syndrome—often arises from the trauma of birth, or other stress or trauma shortly thereafter; it may well be the longest standing, undetected, misunderstood, yet dangerous, condition the person has experienced, since being born. (Not counting genetic factors.)

It is hoped that the methods in this book will help the many who suffer from this syndrome, and that I, or others, can be available for those who need further help. For the methods in this book are still basic techniques; there are more advanced techniques that are not easily depicted this way. And the factors that originally affect the stomach, and the Vagus Nerve, are many and deep, and often require more. But the reader must first make the diet and lifestyle changes described in the first section. They and the basic corrections should help very significantly.

Maybe one day the best toast or wish for a friend's health and longevity will be "May Your Stomach Always Be Down!"

So to all my readers I say...

"May Your Stomach Always Be Down!"

"And May Your Vagus Nerve Always Be In Balance."

Appendix A

SLEEP APNEA:
Silent Pandemic Killer, and Hidden Cause Of Heart Attack *and* Cancer—and *Often Caused by, or Related to, the Hiatal Hernia Syndrome*

This book is the first to explicitly link asthma, *sleep apnea,* the PFO, and other heart conditions, to the HHS or VNI. As sleep apnea is now pandemic, and often still ignored by many or most in the medical or health professions, it is necessary to include this section on the nature, testing, and orthodox and holistic treatments for it.

Possible **symptoms of sleep apnea** include trouble going to, or staying, asleep, or being tired and unrefreshed upon awakening. Being tired or sleepy during the day—including full-blown narcolepsy, and snoring are other possible symptoms, as is waking up gasping. It is a mistake to think that sleep apnea only affects the elderly or middle aged, or the obese.

There are two main types of sleep apnea: Obstructive Sleep Apnea (OSA) and Central Sleep Apnea (CSA). A third type is their combination or Mixed Sleep Apnea (MSD). **Obstructive Sleep Apnea** refers to the closing off of part of the airways in the throat. Snoring is usually heard in sufferers of OSA. Snoring does not always occur, but a close-by snorer can have a decibel level exceeding that of a jet flying 100 feet overhead. The snorer will almost never be able to hear his/her own snoring, but the partner sure can! Many a marriage may have been prevented or terminated due to the decibel levels emitted by the snoring sleep apnea sufferer, and the partner's own ensuing inability to sleep. So saving a marriage can be another reason to get tested and treated.

Central sleep apnea refers to the brain not sufficiently innervating the muscles of respiration, which includes the diaphragm, and abdominal and rib muscles. CSA may be caused by cardiac conditions, including the usually hidden PFO or hole in the heart. The PFO, or other cardiovascular problem, can lead to hypoperfusion of the brain. After a while, it is thought that many people with just OSA eventually also develop the central form. Obstructive sleep apnea can be treated with devices (CPAP or BiPAP) that breathe into sufferers, surgery, dental appliances, and other methods. These other methods can include tongue muscle exercises and advanced energy balancing. Central sleep apnea is treated via the breathing devices, especially BiPAP. SIDS (sudden infant death syndrome) may be a manifestation of sleep apnea—perhaps more likely CSA.

Sleep apnea—by virtue of the low oxygen states induced by obstructive or central sleep apnea—stresses the heart, raises the blood pressure, ages the heart more rapidly, and can cause a heart attack at any time, if the apnic event lasts long enough. Diminished sleep, especially the REM fraction, leads to a sub-optimally functioning brain, which can cause narcolepsy, fatigue, accidents, "mental illness", and other problems.

A 2002 study reported that "On the basis of the average of prevalence estimates from these studies of predominantly white men and women with mean BMI [Body Mass Index] of 25 to 28, we estimate that roughly **1 of every 5 adults has at least mild OSA and 1 of every 15 has at least moderate OSA**." This presumably refers to people in the USA.[14]

A poll taken in the USA in 2005 led to the following conclusion by David M. Hiestand, MD, PhD, et al: "Of the 1,506 respondents, **26%** (31% of men and 21% of women) met the Berlin questionnaire criteria indicating a high risk of OSA. The risk of OSA increased up to age 65 years. A significant number of obese individuals (57%) were at high risk for OSA. Those whose Berlin questionnaire scores indicated a high risk for OSA were more likely to report subjective sleep problems, a negative impact of sleep on quality of life, and a chronic medical condition than those who were at lower risk. Conclusions: **As many as one in four American adults could benefit from evaluation for OSA.** Considering the serious adverse health and quality-of-life consequences of OSA, efforts to expedite diagnosis and treatment are indicated."[15]

In 2012, an important article noted that hypoxia (an inadequate supply of oxygen) that occurs in sleep apnea promotes angiogenesis. This increase in the vascularity is associated with tumor growth. **A 4.8 times higher incidence of cancer mortality may thus be associated with sleep apnea.**[16] Sleep apnea also has increased risk for stroke and diabetes.[17]

Note that it appears that most studies only looked for obstructive sleep apnea and not central sleep apnea. So the percentage, at least in the USA, may be even higher. And the physician-authors are probably being conservative as well. Thus the prevalence for all forms of sleep apnea may be 25%, or more, of adults in some countries. So sleep apnea is pandemic in western society. It is a leading cause of fatigue, brain fatigue and rapid aging.

Predisposing factors for sleep apnea include sinus disease, tonsillectomy, obesity, smoking, alcohol consumption, and as noted, in my opinion, the hiatal hernia syndrome, and also MCS and EMFS. It is important to note that many quite thin people also have sleep apnea. I believe that additional factors can be causative as well and include **hypothyroidism, and micro-organism infection**—such as the very small spirochetes causing Lyme and other diseases. These may get into the brain, or otherwise play a role here. A tendency towards having trigger points can play a role here as well. Sleeping on a memory foam mattress or overlay may help a lot—after it has outgassed for those with MCS. Of course this works both ways. Sleep apnea contributes to causing fibromyalgia and other pain syndromes.

The more problematic central sleep apnea usually does not entail snoring. CSA may be more problematic because there may be less likelihood of the person waking up during an apnic event, as the brain's signals are diminished with CSA, as opposed to OSA where a throat blockage occurs, and the person usually awakens—sometimes gasping.

It sounds innocuous to say "she died peacefully in her sleep." But what if "she" had undiagnosed sleep apnea and could have lived several more years? So if the testing or treatment seems problematic, or if you just don't envision this as a serious problem, imagine this. Someone is coming into your room up to a hundred times an hour, and he goes toward you and places his hands on your throat and chokes you for 30 seconds or longer. Many people who undergo the sleep test are shocked to find that they had serious apnic events, up to a hundred times an hour. What you feel as an inability to go to sleep, is revealed during the test as numerous apnic events. So envision ridding yourself of someone choking you many times each night.

What took place some eight years ago with a client can be instructive. The person had MCS and EMFS. She also reported strange feelings and difficulty during the night—awakening with distress. I told her this could well be sleep apnea and that she should immediately schedule a test and get treatment if she has sleep apnea. Her husband replied that she did not snore. To this, I replied that that could mean she has the even more problematic central sleep apnea, and again I implored her to get tested ASAP. She replied that she had MCS and EMFS, and it was too difficult. I nonetheless implored her again. She did not schedule any type of testing, and died just a few weeks later in her sleep. She was in her forties.

Yes both the testing and treatment can be difficult for someone with MCS and/or EMFS. Indeed **sensitivity to chemicals or EMF can be part of the cause of sleep apnea.** As far as chemicals are concerned, you can be reacting to fragrance, formaldehyde, mold or other things in the room or bed—both at home or at the sleep center. Regarding EMF, you may be reacting to the AC current in the room, or nearby towers, WiFi, or even the coils in your mattress set can absorb and re-radiate radio waves or microwaves.

The **kindling effect** may play a large role in sleep problems. Just looking at TV or computer monitor screens can lead to hyper brain states. Indeed I have had clients report back, after I had tested them, that not only sleep, but their asthma or hypoglycemia was better when they avoided TV and the internet. Some people also have hyperacusis and must avoid sounds to feel and sleep better. Again the PFO, or other cardiovascular problem, may be causing hypoperfusion in the brain. Also allergic, or porphyric, reactions to foods such as wheat, sugar, caffeine, or others, also cause hyper states in many people.

The testing of sleep apnea is called a polysomnograph. The person reports to a sleep center for 10-12 hours. After a briefing and orientation to the room, the subject is "wired up" with sensors. These sensors may go on the chest, legs (looking for restless leg syndrome), face, and throat. Sensors on the head will be part of an EEG to measure brain waves, and there will also be an ECG (electrocardiogram) run throughout the test. Real time monitoring and video recording also takes place. Because of the cost, distance, and the different environment of the sleep centers, home testing is also in the early stages. Here the sensors and recording devices may be picked up or shipped to the patient.

During the test, if the sleep technician sees—or the sensors indicate—significant sleep apnea and/or concomitant medical problems, he or she may come in to the room, and put the subject on an air pressure machine. When this occurs, the optimum settings for inhalation and exhalation can be gauged. Different types of nasal or nasal/mouth attachments can also be tested for efficacy. Sometimes—due to insufficient sleep during the test—a second one may be desired.

If both a sleep center and home testing are not available to you in your region or country, the following can be used to help determine the possibility of your having sleep apnea. Medical oxygen suppliers also often can provide a **home recorded pulse oximetry** kit. This entails a pulse oximeter placed overnight on your fingertip and attached to a recorder. Episodes of hypoxia may be evidence of apnic events—especially if other heart and lung diseases have been ruled out. Pulse rate is also recorded this way. It may be a good idea for sufferers of any chronic illness to purchase their own pulse oximeter as these now sell for under $50, about one-tenth of what they were a dozen years ago when I first bought one for myself and clients. The oximeter shines an LED light through the fingernail and detects the oxygen level on the hemoglobin of red blood cells. Overnight pulse oximetry, of course, cannot detect such things as insufficient REM [rapid eye movement] sleep.

There is a very significant difference between the two types of air pressure machines available—**CPAP and BiPAP. CPAP denotes Continuous Positive Airway Pressure.** CPAP devices have one continuous level, or one maximum level, of air pressure—presumably optimally determined from analyzing the polysomnograph data. CPAP was invented by Sydney, Australia physician, Dr. Colin Sullivan in 1980. Prior to that, tracheotomy was actually employed for (severe) sleep apnea. Sullivan was a SIDS researcher.

BiPAP refers to Bi-level Positive Airway Pressure. The "bi-level" means that two different settings are used with these devices. The higher level refers to the maximum pressure the machine can emit when it senses you are—*or should be*—breathing in, and the lower level is the device's maximum pressure when it senses you are breathing out. The higher air pressure is needed to force air past blocked airways. Some of these devices can sense if they need to emit their maximal pressures during inspiration and expiration, and they may emit a pressure less than their maxima if that is not needed at that moment. Even in patients without sleep apnea, BiPAP machines are now being used for COPD, pneumonia, asthma, and heart failure.

The difference between CPAP and BiPAP devices is evident during the exhalation phase. With BiPAP, this pressure is significantly less than its pressure during inhalation, so the person does not have to breathe out against the higher pressure when it is not needed to do so. The CPAP device has only the one level, though more recent CPAP devices may have some (sensor controlled) variability capability. The point is that it can be an unnecessary struggle to breath out against the machine for some or many. The elderly, asthmatics, the obese and people with other conditions can have difficulty with CPAP. Indeed it is hoped here that CPAP will eventually be eliminated and everyone who tries these devices gets a BiPAP. It is estimated that about 50% of people who try CPAP discontinue its use. Many of these people do not get other treatments, and so are at great risk. Perhaps if only BiPAP were used, the 50% figure would go down. If you get a CPAP or BiPAP device make sure to get it with a heated humidifier. With this, the air first passes over a container of water, which itself can be heated. This prevents dry and/or cold air from entering your lungs, which could cause problems. People with asthma or RAD (reactive airways disease), or other medical conditions will not do well with dry or cold air. Inexpensive bacterial filters can also be added in the air hose line.

The CPAP or BiPAP machines themselves can be problematic for sufferers of MCS or EMFS. To lessen the sound level, there is foam in the machines that needs to outgas for the chemically sensitive. Likewise the full mouth and nose coverings can have numerous chemicals. If just a nasal cannula can be used, silicone cannulae are made that usually are well tolerated in those with MCS. Timely outgassing of the full mouth cannulae and the machines themselves should help. The machines, of course, emit their own EMF. But that intensity falls off with the square of distance, and a longer hose can be used. The machine could also be shielded and surrounded by aluminum foil for the very EMF sensitive. Some people report correcting the chemical or electromagnetic problems with their sleep room corrected or ameliorated their "insomnia."

Another possible treatment for OSA is an oral appliance. Specially trained dentists can make a molding and create a dental appliance that facilitates keeping the airway in the back of the throat open during sleep, thus preventing or reducing apnic events. This does not help central sleep apnea. People with significant sinus disease may not be able to use CPAP or BiPAP. I knew someone who had nasal surgery and because of this when she tried to use CPAP, the air went into her stomach, not her lungs, and she got a dental appliance.

The Buteyko system advocates report that just **taping the lips closed during sleep**—to prevent low CO_2 status (hypocapnia)—can improve sleep.

Surgery for OSD is also available, and there are at least three variations. These are traditional (scalpel) surgery, radio wave surgery and laser surgery. The first probably occurs most often. The last—laser surgery—is probably the most expensive but is said to yield the best results and quickest recovery, though insurance companies often only reimburse for the first option, and then only if the pressure devices cannot be used or tolerated. With the last two options, radio waves or laser beams burn away some throat tissue. Note that with all three types of throat surgery, some people report that throat tissue grew back. And I know that those who do neural therapy injections would not advise the massive creation of scar tissue. But I do know people who did well with laser surgery.

There is clearly a **hiatal hernia connection**. I have had clients tell me that upon following my advise, and elevating the top of their bed and/or sleeping on a wedge, their "insomnia" vanished or improved. Obviously making the diet and lifestyle changes herein would be a good idea. As would doing the simple, self-help corrections for the hernia, diaphragm and vagus nerve. Before sleep is a good time to do these corrections.

Now one of the mainstays of hiatal hernia treatment is to not eat for several hours before going to sleep. This can be problematic for those with reactive hypoglycemia or porphyria. Hypoglycemics and/or porphyrics might crash in a few hours and so will tend to want to eat just before going to sleep. This may then cause apnic events because of the hiatal hernia. People who get up a few hours after going to sleep and can't go back to sleep, and may also be hungry or agitated at that time, may be hypoglycemic and/or porphyric. Taking Vitamin B_6 before sleep can also cause some people to get up a few hours later, and be unable to go back to sleep.

There are additional items that may improve sleep and also ameliorate chronic pain syndromes. First I will describe the little known **Eeman screens.** Leon Ernest Eeman was a British WWI pilot who crashed shortly after taking off, and was left in a disabled state. He suffered from constant, severe pain, which also prevented him from sleeping. His doctors told him it was hopeless. He began to study everything available to try to help himself. He created copper plates that when placed in certain positions on or under his body cured his pain and sleep problems. The underlying basis for this can variously be called polarity, or maybe Tibetan energy flows or figure 8 energy flow. So perhaps

Eeman came across some ancient eastern wisdom. Kinesiologists also put the body in a figure 8 position to facilitate this energy flow. But the copper screens apparently significantly increase the proper energy flow in the body—whatever that may be.

Some people have reported a duplication of Eeman's results of pain or insomnia cessation. You can search online for companies that make copper Eeman screens. These involve a copper screen attached to a tubular copper rod that is held in the hand. A screen is placed under the head and that one is attached to a copper rod that will be held by the left hand. At the same time a second copper screen is placed under the base of the spine (coccyx), and that one is attached to a copper rod, which is held by the right hand. The feet must be such that the left foot is on top of the right foot. This can be problematic for those with arthritis or obesity.

A variation of the Eeman circuit is called the **Lindemann Symmetrical Circuit,** and it may be a more powerful improvement. Three sets of copper screens are used. One set is for the head and the coccyx (screens on both ends), and the other two sets are for each foot with the other end being held by the opposite hand. The feet can be kept apart with this set-up. The feet screens, at least, should come with attached straps. Note that one acupuncture method for people with poor circulation in the extremities is to needle certain points on the feet and hands simultaneously. This may work similarly. But here there are no needles, no electricity, only the body's own energies apparently being properly directed or re-directed.

Another method that may afford improved sleep and/or pain reduction is the use of a **FIR (far infrared) heating pad**. This does involve AC current and so may not be for those with certain problems such as EMFS, Mast Cell Disease and others. But as with the Eeman screens, some people report a deep calm coming over them in minutes that helps reduce pain and/or leads to sleep. I have tried both these methods (and have no connections to any of their manufacturers), and can attest that they can quickly afford deep relaxation, but were not curative of anything for me. Again this is not a substitute for a sleep study and other treatment if the problem is moderate or severe.

Drug treatment for insomnia can be very dangerous if sleep apnea is what is really occurring. That is because the drugs may artificially "knock out" the sufferer to the extent that he or she may not wake up during an apnic event.

Supplements for insomnia have been very popular for decades. These have included tryptophan, 5HTP, and melatonin. For some people these work fine. People with asthma or porphyria may not tolerate any of those. Often better tolerated—even for (hidden) porphyrics—can be **GABA or the newer form, PharmaGABA**. GABA is an amino acid and inhibitory neurotransmitter found in the brain, and the PharmaGABA form better crosses the blood-brain barrier and is taken in smaller amounts. It can provide a very natural calmness and sometimes sleepiness. For chronic pain sufferers I also note that recently **D-Phenylalanine** became available—not the D'L form, but pure D-Phenylalanine. This appears to be far more effective for pain and can also aid sleep. But again no supplement should be a substitute for getting a polysomnograph if sleep apnea is suspected. And all supplements should ideally first be kinesiologically tested.

Sleep may also be facilitated by placing a cold gel pack on top of the head—and/or cooling down the room. The gel pack is stored in your freezer for use when you have anxiety, insomnia or similar problems. This may also help with pain, flushing, and even respiratory and circulatory problems. The ancient Greeks knew some things better than do physicians today. They coined the term *hothead* and sought ways to cool down the *hot head* in people with hyperactivity or anxiety. If mild insomnia is present, try this. According to oriental medicine, flushing may occur because some aspects of Chi may not be flowing to the extremities and builds up and overheats the head and face. Western medicine might say or find that blood and/or lymph flow is reduced to the extremities, and again flushing can result. There may be underlying cardiac problems, and/or such things as reaction to MSG or certain foods ongoing.

While the head may be overheated, the extremities may be too cold. Some people will sleep better while wearing socks and gloves. Organic cotton may be best for the chemically sensitive. If tolerated, FIR socks and FIR gloves are now available, as are FIR blankets and FIR mattress covers. These reflect the body's heat back to the wearer. On the other hand, some people, when ill or agitated, have very irritable skin and may prefer to sleep totally nude. They may not want to wear any clothes at all during the day as well. Irritable skin while agitated is unfortunately considered by some to be a psychiatric disorder—as depicted by the Billy Chenowith character in *Six Feet Under*—but is understood by this author to be a manifestation of **mast cell disease**. MCD, in my opinion, is another hidden cause of the explosion of sleep disorders presently.

There are mouth/throat/tongue exercises that may reduce obstructive sleep apnea by strengthening airway muscles.

1. Press your tongue flat against the floor of the mouth, and brush the top and sides with a toothbrush. Repeat brushing 5 times. Perform several times a day.

2. Press length of tongue to the roof of the mouth, and hold for 2-3 minutes—once daily.

3. Place a finger into one side of mouth. Hold the finger against cheek while pulling cheek muscle in at same time. Repeat 8 times, then rest and alternate sides. Repeat 3 times.

4. Purse your lips as if to kiss. Hold your lips tightly together, and move them up and to the right; then up and to the left 10 times. Repeat 2-3 times during the day.

Advanced kinesiology methods I devised are far too involved to present here. I have created a mode or test for sleep apnea and then use the advanced method to balance as much as possible for it, if it tests positive. All the kinesiological modes I have devised—including for sleep problems, PFO, porphyria and other imbalances—were correlated with positive medical test results. Every person's advanced balance is different, and the word "cure" is never used here. I still advise everyone who suspects they might have sleep apnea to get the overnight sleep study, or at least overnight pulse oximetry, and to undergo one of the treatments if significant apnea is found.

Having a CPAP, or better BiPAP, around is a good idea. BiPAP machines, we saw above, are even being used for respiratory and cardiac emergency or failure. A prescription for a device will list its parameters. For example, a BiPAP might be written up with the make and model of the device desired for the patient, and the diagnosis, and say something like 17/12. This would refer to its two main settings. The higher number is the setting for inspiration or IPAP, and the lower number is the setting for exhalation or EPAP. (The pressure units are "millimeters of mercury.") A CPAP device has just the one parameter, and might say "14 mm.".

All too many of both orthodox and holistic medical practitioners act as if they believe their role is confined to dispensing pills and many do not consider testing and treating for many causative factors, including possible underlying sleep apnea which is pandemic now. If one out of four adults has sleep apnea in general, it may imply that a significantly higher percentage of the people who go to holistic practitioners have some form of sleep apnea—due to the type of complaints often presented. Yet many holistic physicians, I have found, do not know how to write a prescription for the test, nor how to read the simple report conclusions or how to prescribe for a CPAP or BiPAP device.

Untreated sleep apnea plays a role in causing or exacerbating accidents, chronic fatigue, brain fog, fibromyalgia and other pain syndromes, hypertension, heart disease, more rapid aging, and even cancer we have recently seen. Of course, death can occur at any time as well. Common signs are trouble going to or staying asleep, snoring, tiredness during the day and others

If you have sleep apnea, get some form of treatment for it soon. Due to the seriousness of this condition, the decision to undergo a sleep study—if you have the symptoms—should be made immediately. Clearly it should not be a decision…to sleep on.

With a nod to the Bard, I say that one of our goals might be: "To sleep, perchance to dream…*better still to wake up anew and with vitality.*"

BIBLIOGRAPHY

1.*Porphyria: The Ultimate Cause of Common, Chronic or Environmental Illnesses. With Diet, Supplement and Energy Balancing, 2nd Ed*.   Rochlitz, Steven. ISBN: 0-945262-59-0 2011, Cottonwood, AZ. [See inside back cover.]

2. *Hiatal Hernia Syndrome: Insidious Link to Major Illness, 6th Ed.* Baroody, Theodore J., Holographic Health Press. 1998.

3. *The Hole in the Heart—Which One out of Three of us Have.* Rochlitz, Steven. Cottonwood, AZ . [See inside back cover.]

4. http://www.france24.com/en/20090727-sarkozy-leaves-hospital-after-night-under-observation--health-french-president-france-vagus-nerve

5. Simons DG, Travell JG, Simons LS. *Travell & Simon's Myofascial pain and Dysfunction The Trigger Point Manual Vol. I. 2nd Ed.* Lippincott, Williams & Wilkins. 1999.

6. Stiennon, O. Arthur. *The Longitudinal Muscle in Esophageal Disease.* Radiology Publishing. 1995.

7. *Allergies and Candida: with the Physicist's Rapid Solution,54th Edition*. Rochlitz, Steven. ISBN: 0-945262-48-5 2012. [See inside back cover.]

8. Huang, M.Z., Huo, L.Q. The effect of acupuncture needle stimulation of the phrenic nerve in resuscitation during respiratory arrest. *Am J Acupuncture*. 1992; 20:223-228.

9. Philibert HH. *The Anatomy of Pain. Specific Injection Therapy*. 2000 Metairie, LA

10. Prudden, Bonnie. *Myotherapy: Bonnie Prudden's Complete Guide To Pain-Free Living*. Ballantine Books. New York. 1985.

11. *The Breath of Life*. Ellis, George. 1993. Newcastle. Van Nuys, CA

12. Task Force. Standards of Heart Rate Variability. *Circulation*. 93:1059

13. Porge, Stephen. Cardiac Vagal Tone: A Physiological Index of Stress. *Neuroscience and Biobehavioral Reviews*. 19/2:225-233

14. Terry Young, Paul E. Peppard and Daniel J. Gottlieb. Epidemiology of Obstructive Sleep Apnea: A Population Health Perspective. *Am. J. Respir. Crit. Care Med*. May 1, 2002 vol. 165 no. 9 1217-1239.
http://ajrccm.atsjournals.org/content/165/9/1217.full

15. David M. Hiestand, et al. Prevalence of Symptoms and Risk of Sleep Apnea in the US Population: Results From the National Sleep Foundation Sleep in America 2005 Poll. *Chest Journal*. September 2006, Vol 130, No. 3.
http://journal.publications.chestnet.org/article.aspx?articleid=1084669

16. F. Javier Nieto, et al. Sleep-disordered Breathing and Cancer Mortality: Results from the Wisconsin Sleep Cohort Study. *Am. J. Respir. Crit. Care Med.* 2012; 186: 190-194.
http://ajrccm.atsjournals.org/content/186/2/190.abstract

17.http://www.cbsnews.com/8301-504763_162-57438371-10391704/people-with-severe-sleep-apnea-five-times-more-likely-to-die-from-cancer-study-shows/

Index

Hiccups: 16
Hoarseness: 16
Homeopathic Remedies: 28, 48
Hypertension: 16, 21, 28, 65
Hypocapnia: 32, 34, 48, 60
Hypoglycemia: 17, 29, 57
Hypotension: 16, 17
Hypothyroidism: 55
Inflammation: 28
Infraspinatus: 5, 41
Insomnia: 17, 60-63
Kidney: 17, 18
Kindling: 57
Kinesiology: 24-6, 36, 43-5, 64
Lindemann Circuit: 62
Lyme Disease: 55
Mast Cell Disease: 44, 62, 64
Mercury: 14, 27, 30, 31, 65
MSG: 27, 63
Multiple Chemical Sensitivities
(MCS): 14, 23, 35, 46, 55-6, 59
Nausea: 16
Neck: 17, 35, 49
Nightshades: 23
Nitric oxide: 19
Norepinephrine: 19
Numbness: 17, 20
Obesity: 17, 29, 55, 62
Obstructive Sleep Apnea (OSA):
53-56, 60, 64, 66
PFO (Patent Foramen Ovale): 15,
16, 53, 54, 57, 65
Pain: 16, 17, 20, 29, 35, 40, 55,
61, 62, 63, 65, 68
Panic: 16, 30
Parasympathetic Nerv.System: 18
Pectoralis muscle: 40
Philibert, Harry: 40, 41, 68
PharmaGABA: 48, 63
Phrenic nerve: 35, 49, 68
Polysomnograph: 57, 58, 63
Porphyria: 39

Pregnancy: 17, 26
Prostate: 17
Prudden, Bonnie: 42, 68
Pulse Oximetry: 58, 65
Pull-Down (stomach): 21, 42
Reactive airways disease: 59
Reflexology: 5, 26, 46, 47
Regurgitation: 16
Respiratory collapse: 35
Sarkozy, Nicolas: 20, 67
Schatzki's (LES) ring: 25, 26
Shoulder: 16, 41, 42
SIDS: 54, 58
Sinus Disease: 55, 60
Sleep apnea: 9, 10, 14, 17, 53-66
          Mouth exercises: 64
Smoking: 55
Spirochetes: 55
Stiennon, O. Arthur: 26, 67
Stomach: throughout
Stress: 17, 19-24, 32, 33, 34, 43,
46, 50-52, 67
Supraventricular tachycardia: 16,
20
Surgery: 50, 54, 60, 61
Swallowing Difficulty: 26, 49
Sympathetic Nervous System: 18
Tachycardia: 16, 20, 25
Thyroid: 17, 24, 34, 45, 55
Thimerosal: 30
TMJ: 17, 45
Tonsillectomy: 27, 55
TransCranial Doppler (test): 16
Trigger Point(s): 20, 21, 23, 27,
32, 40-42, 55, 68
Ulcer: 16, 28
Vagus Nerve Imbalance (VNI):
throughout
Vasoactive Intestinal
          Polypeptide (VIP): 27
Viruses: 31
Wedge (bed): 23, 61
Xiphoid process: 42

Steven Rochlitz, PhD has taught both Physics and Kinesiology at three Universities in the USA. He has taught his Human Ecology Balancing Sciences [HEBS] Seminars, across four continents. He is the author of ten books, and numerous articles. Clients have come to see him from five continents. Phone, in-person consultations, and seminars may possibly be available with the author.

Also by the Author:

The Hole in the Heart, Which 1 out of 3 of us Has, and Blood-Brain Barrier Permeability In Chronic & Environmental Illness. Copyright 2012. Steven Rochlitz, PhD. *The crucial sister book to this one.* ISBN: 978-0-945262-62-0 $22.00 each. 110 pages, 16 illustrations. Shipping: $5.00. or $10.00 to overseas.

Porphyria: The Ultimate Cause of Common, Chronic or Environmental Illnesses. With Diet, Supplement and Energy Balancing, 2nd Edition Steven Rochlitz, PhD ISBN: 0-945262-53-1 $40..00 plus $7.00 shipping, $15. to overseas.. *This book contains many hidden factors that may predispose the Vagus Nerve to imbalance.*

Allergies and Candida: with the Physicist's Rapid Solution, 5th Edition *by Steven Rochlitz PhD, Foreword by John Wright M.D.* ISBN 0-945262-48-5 272 Pages, Illustrated. 2011. $30.00 plus $7.00 (in the USA) for air mail, $13.00 overseas. For learning how to overcome allergies, Candidiasis, Parasitosis, chronic fatigue, fibromyalgia, environmental illness, chronic illness and learning disorders. Everyone with these problems has many food sensitivities and overgrowths of microorganisms. Learn how 80-90% of "Candida" is something else—perhaps protozoan parasitosis, perhaps.... Contains four chapters on self-help, illustrated kinesiological techniques

Supercharge Your Heart In Seconds: The Rochlitz Discoveries for Anti-Aging, Heart Health, Blood Pressure, Maximum Athletic Performance and M.S. Steven Rochlitz, PhD **146 pages $25.00 + shipping. ISBN:** 0-945262-60-4. Foreword by Chief Justice Charles Springer, Former title: ***Why Do Music Conductors Live Into Their 90's?***

Hiatal Hernia Syndrome/Vagus Nerve Imbalance: With Illustrated Corrections, Third Edition Steven Rochlitz, PhD. 72 pages, Illustrated. $20.00 each. Shipping: $5.00. ($8.00 overseas.)

Quantity orders for this Hiatal Hernia Syndrome/Vagus Nerve Imbalance book are available. Help your friends, family, patients, students. Inquire.

Three Advanced H.E.B.S. Seminar Manuals are available in their respective HEBS Seminars. Human Ecology Balancing Sciences Seminars include Prof. Rochlitz' breakthrough kinesiology testing & balancing methods. Consultations & seminars may be available on a limited basis. If you wish to be a trainee, volunteer, or possibly a certified successor, contact us. Serious inquiries please.

All prices subject to change.

Steven Rochlitz, PhD
P.O. Box 2154 Cottonwood, Arizona 86326 USA
(928) 649-2116
www.wellatlast.com
info@wellatlast.com